Gordon Inkeles' *The Art of Sensual Massage* demystified the practice of massage. It was an instant best-seller and remains just as popular eight years later. *The New Massage* offers a complete body massage, with emphasis on those massage techniques that complement exercise. Whatever type of exercise you take you will find that the skills that *The New Massage* encourages will increase endurance, lower fatigue levels, relax and soothe aching muscles and leave you feeling totally rejuvenated.

The New Massage explores special problems: muscle hardening, cramps, sprains, ankle and foot injuries and includes a special section on massage as a drugless therapy that can cure nervous tension and stress, headaches and stomach disorders.

Illustrated throughout with many photographs and diagrams, the book is a joy to travel through and it is written with the same blend of knowledge, humour and warmth that made *The Art of Sensual Massage* so popular.

Also by Gordon Inkeles
THE ART OF SENSUAL MASSAGE
(with Murray Todris)

Also by Gordon Inkeles

THE ART OF SENSUAL MASSAGE
(*with Murray Todris*)

First published in the United States of America by Perigee
Books, a division of G. P. Putman's Sons.
First published in Great Britain by Unwin Paperbacks 1981.
Reprinted 1984

This edition based on the original book design and illustration
by Jon Goodchild.
American usage and spelling have been retained.

UNWIN PAPERBACKS
40 Museum Street, London WC1A 1LU

British Library Cataloguing in Publication Data

Inkeles, Gordon
    The new massage.
    1. Massage
    613.7'9   RA780.5

    ISBN 0–04–613043–8

Printed in Hong Kong by
Dah Hua Printing Press Co. Ltd.

Skin Lore

The tactile sense is the original sense, the first sense developed by the most ancient single-celled creatures on earth. For 3 billion years they have lived in a dark, utterly silent world where every-thing that is known is felt. In human beings the tactile sense is the primary sense.

Apart from the brain itself, the skin is the body's most complex organ. Any square inch of it contains hundreds of pleasure, pain, pressure, heat, and cold receptors. In the same square inch you can find fifteen feet of blood vessels and about seventy-two feet of nerves. Skin is the

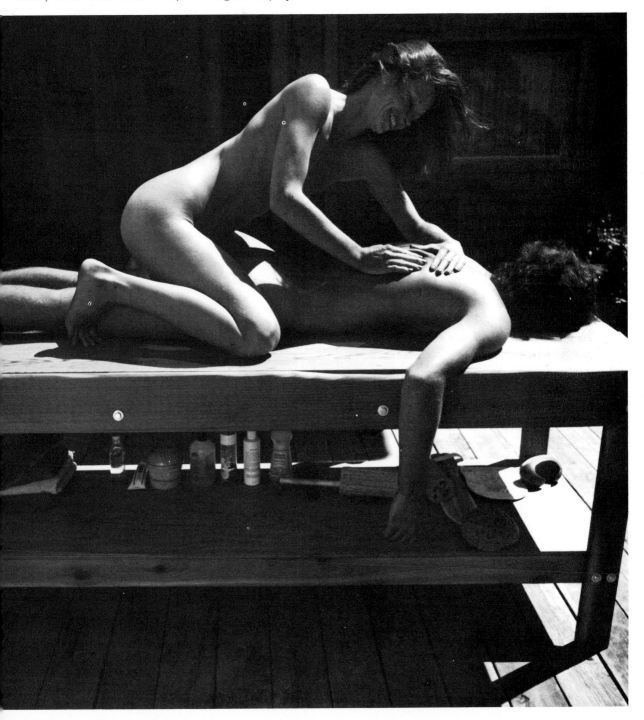

"eye" of the nervous system. Every massage movement will contact it directly. Its thickness can vary from about one-fiftieth of an inch on the eyelids to as much as one-third of an inch on the palms and soles. Throughout the body the skin has three layers which fit together snugly via countless ridges and valleys. The two inner layers are covered with a rich carpet of blood vessels, glands, nerves, and fat lobules. Part of the exposed top layer is made of a horny material that is actually dead skin cells. These dead cells can clog the pores and keep the skin from feeling and breathing naturally. Part of the exhilaration that follows a good bath comes from discarding some of this dead, horny layer of skin.

Puritanical attitudes toward the body are nowhere more apparent than in the bathing habits common to most Americans. People bathe merely to remove dirt from their bodies, not to feel anything. We have a nation obsessed with gratification that ignores the most basic sense and the body's largest organ.

Since all massage movements affect the skin, the aim of the premassage bath is to clean the skin far more thoroughly than ordinary soap-and-water bathing. The idea is to bring the skin to a point where it can feel and then stimulate it so it will feel. By doing this, you increase the tactile possibilities for the entire massage, and no matter how much massage your partner has experienced, he will notice a difference after a premassage bath. Even before the massage begins, your partner becomes relaxed and totally aware of his body.

Studies of very old people all over the world reveal one factor common to all of them: Throughout their lives they sweat copiously every day. This curious fact, often cited by sauna enthusiasts, would seem to imply that the oceans of sweat generated after fifteen minutes in a sauna can actually extend one's life. But the kind of sweating these old folks do is usually the result of good old-fashioned manual labor, still popular in those parts of the world where leisure time is scarce and exercise for its own sake has not yet become fashionable. The idea that it is healthful or even generally beneficial to roast your body, which is mostly water, at temperatures very near the boiling

point of water is certainly debatable. Many people bolt from the sauna in four or five minutes, hearts racing, feeling slightly dizzy, and doubting their own senses. Wasn't this supposed to be a relaxing experience? For some people it definitely is; you may not be one of them. One of the most important considerations in any bath is the way one feels afterward.

Saunas, Jacuzzis, and hot tubs are expensive to set up and use huge amounts of energy. (If you already have one and want to use it with massage, please see "How Bath Temperatures Affect the Body," page 26). A body shampoo costs practically nothing and uses less energy than a shower. It will leave your partner feeling absolutely wonderful without using 800 gallons of hot water, a specially designed redwood room, or high-speed electrical devices. During a body shampoo, you become directly involved with the bath by using your own hands, thus establishing the kind of close physical contact you will be sharing during the massage. The body shampoo will do even more for your skin than a sauna, without taxing the heart or making you sweat. If massage is your aim, it's better to sweat and exercise your heart when you exercise your body. Use the body shampoo to get your partner cleaner than he's ever been in his life. It's the ideal introduction to the world of massage—you can lie back and do absolutely nothing but feel. For most people the experience of being bathed becomes a dreamy sort of return to early childhood, the last time anyone touched or bathed their entire body.

The most important aspect of communal bathing is simply the experience of being bathed by another person. This is easiest on a bath table, but if you don't have space, you can certainly improvise in your own bathtub or shower. Use soap and a flexible

shower spray to direct water to specific parts of your partner's body. A shampoo brush, loofah, or bath mitt will loosen the dead surface layer of skin and stimulate the growth of new cells. These simple tools leave your partner's skin relaxed and glowing the first time you use them. Cover the whole body with soft round strokes. You can use pressures on the back and legs which are virtually impossible for an individual bathing alone.

Almost as delightful as being bathed by another person and equally foreign to the experience of most Americans is the exotic sensation of being oiled. A very light bath oil can be prepared simply by mixing one part almond with two parts sesame seed oil. Add a bit of lemon to restore the skin's slightly acidic pH. Bath oil replaces natural skin oils that are always lost to soap and water. Oil the skin after a bath and salt rub.

The Salt Rub

Salt rubs are not for the timid or extremely sensitive. They are massively stimulating and, for those who enjoy them, absolutely indispensable. If your partner has a lot of body hair, this is one way to amplify the cleansing action of a body shampoo substantially. The effects of a brief salt rub are immediately apparent and visible. Skin reddening all over the body gives direct evidence of the enormous potential this treatment has as a circulation stimulant. Beyond that, the salt rub acts as a kind of general tonic for the entire body. The salt's mildly abrasive effect will remove all the skin debris you may have missed during the body shampoo and leave your partner tingling.

You need to moisten your partner's body slightly with a damp washcloth to temper the abrasive action of the salt on skin. For the same reason it's best to dampen the salt a bit before you begin. Use coarse salt if possible.

Take a moment to be sure there are no cuts or tender spots anywhere on your partner's body. Salt will irritate them and spoil the effect of the rub. Go easy on the face. Avoid the area around the eyes and mouth.

Once you've moistened the whole body, cover your washcloth with a moderately thick layer of salt. Salt, like massage oil, is more easily controlled when you add it to your hand and avoid dumping it onto the skin. Any rubbing that precedes a massage should imitate the rhythms of massage. Try to avoid jerky scrubbing motions on broad expanses

Hot Towels

of the body like the torso and back. The salt rub will be far more effective if you work over your partner's body with vigorous, even, circular strokes. Use the entire flat surface of your hands. Press down and circle with the washcloth while your free hand circles against the skin. Pressures should be about equal. When you've covered every part of the body with at least three vigorous circles, wash the salt off with warm water, and dry your partner.

One sad consequence of living with high stress levels is that a great many people walk around with cold hands and feet. The best way to warm them up along with the rest of the body is with large soft hot towels. You can warm towels by placing them inside a large paper bag and putting it in the oven for ten minutes at 200 degrees. As long as the paper bag isn't exposed to an open flame, it will not burn and your towels will be warm and perfectly dry. If you are fortunate enough to have a towel large enough to reach from head to toe, you can cover your partner's body with a single movement. Working with smaller towels, begin at the feet and overlap the

towels until the body is covered. Whatever size, the towels should go down with one long sweeping motion. Everything that touches your partner during the massage, whether it be your hands, your hair, your knee, or a hot towel, becomes a part of the massage. Because your partner will experience the massage with his eyes closed, the tactile sense is exquisitely sensitized. To help establish the mood, use the same speed and rhythm in laying down the hot towels that you will use later on the legs and arms.

When your partner's entire body is covered, from scalp to toes, pat the towel gently so that it conforms to the outlines of the arms, legs, and torso. This luxurious sensation of being pressed and patted prepares your partner for the warm, infinitely relaxing experience that is about to begin.

Leave the towels on for about five minutes. When you're ready to remove them, pull the bottom edge of the towel slowly and evenly until the top of the towel gradually breaks contact with your partner's toes.

Preparing for Massage

Preparing for Massage

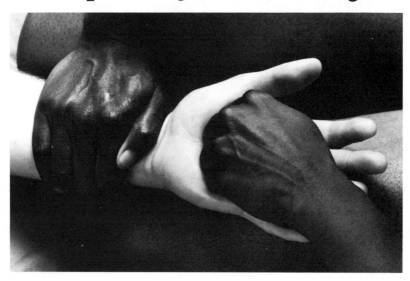

Since massage reaches so many of the senses at once, there should be no interruptions or distractions while you work. The experience is so relaxing and pleasurable that your partner has the chance to yield and become utterly sensitized. Something similar happens to audiences during any serious theatrical effort, and that's why actors don't interrupt a performance to rearrange sets or accept phone calls.

If you view massage as a theatrical situation, you can arrange your place so that very little will distract you or your partner during the experience. Of course, it's not always possible to massage where there are no distractions at all. It's worthwhile, though, to make every effort to quiet things down around your massage area. The obvious distractions to consider right away are ones that might force you to abandon the massage altogether. Make sure that children are cared for and that you're not expecting company. Can you manage to live without phone calls for a few hours? Do you have demanding pets that are likely to bound into the massage area without warning? Your partner will experience the massage with eyes closed, and this, of course, intensifies all the other senses. You may take for granted automatic appliances that switch on and off, television programs in the next room, and the smell of food cooking. Don't expect your partner to miss any of this. Sounds and smells that are routinely shut out can dominate your partner's consciousness during massage. If you're working in a crowded environment where it's difficult to control all these factors, you can provide your own sounds and scents. Choose sounds that your partner likes. You might want to look through a record collection, choose a radio station, or merely open a window to let in the sound of falling rain. Scents are discussed on page 29.

change the course of Western medical thought by incorporating ancient Chinese health principles.

Elsewhere in the East shrewd businessmen have adroitly capitalized on the West's imperfect understanding of acupuncture. They insist that the human body is a living machine which is covered with exotic little pressure points. Once these points are pushed (by fingertips which are several hundred times wider than the point of an acupuncture needle), magical things begin to happen all over the body. Developed and refined in Japan a few years ago, this concept has found a huge audience with Western button lovers, who secretly believe all things Eastern must be 4,000 years old and shrouded in a peculiar mystical aura that cannot be penetrated by the logic-bound Western mind.

Immensely successful pressure point schools have already been franchised throughout Japan and are beginning to catch on here in the United States. Graduates of these schools combine basic massage techniques with aggressive finger poking to the soft, relaxed inner tissues. The resulting pain levels around vital organs are often so great that speech is momentarily impossible. But if speech were possible, the victim might remind his smug tormentor that the human body is not, alas, covered with ubiquitous little push buttons like the dashboard of a Toyota.

Referred Pain

Influencing the health of internal organs with massage requires only a basic understanding of how the nervous system operates. The entire body is controlled by the brain via the nerves. Virtually all the beneficial effects of massage are directly related to changes in the nervous system. Soothe the nerves that supply the liver, and the arteries of the liver dilate.

Most of the internal organs are supplied by nerves that branch at the spinal cord and surface just above the organ itself, but there are a few notable exceptions you should deal with in the course of a complete body massage. Although the heart is primarily supplied by nerves from the spine, heart trouble is usually signaled by pain radiating down the left arm. This phenomenon is called referred pain, and it marks an important nervous connection. Masseurs recognize that because pain from the heart is felt in the left arm it's worthwhile to massage that arm whenever you're working on the heart. The same nerves that carry pain can be used to transmit pleasure. Referred pain centers will be discussed periodically throughout the text. Use them to reach inside the body and soothe the vital organs.

Sleepers

Occasionally, someone will surprise you by falling asleep. One of the most unfortunate effects of accumulated stress is that people eventually reach the point where total relaxation becomes a fond memory. Even during sleep itself, back and shoulder muscles remain somewhat tense and exhaustion takes the place of relaxation. For these people, getting through the long days and nights becomes a kind of grim ordeal, one that often ends abruptly five minutes after massage begins, when they fall into a deep, blissful sleep. This sudden drifting away can be somewhat disconcerting if you're not ready for it because it seems as though your partner has abandoned the massage altogether. On the contrary, sleep is a sign that you have broken through what may be years of accumulated tension.

Since absolutely nothing is required of your partner during a massage except relaxation, you can continue what you were doing because it's working. You're not massaging the conscious mind; you're massaging the body. As you stroke and knead, you'll notice that people rarely move at all during massage sleep. If you finish at the end of the day, you might want to let your partner sleep on until the next morning. (See "Insomnia," page 177.)

Nutrition, Exercise, and Massage

Many Americans, citizens of the world's most abundant food supplier, are seriously worried that they may not be getting their money's worth at the market. So many diet books have attacked modern food processing that all canned, refined or frozen products suddenly appear dangerous and wholly lacking in nutritive value. Nervous purists go even further and deplore the use of anything sweet, salty, spicy or fattening until nearly every dish is regarded with the same dismay that Socrates must have felt for his final cup of hemlock.

How many "health conscious" Americans are afraid of their food when they sit down to the dinner table (while half the world has no dinner or table)? You are what you eat, argues the purist, as he rejects yet another sumptuous dish and begins the familiar lecture on poisons and toxins. Guilt masquerading as health awareness brings stress to the dinner table and guarantees an utterly joyless meal. For thousands of years human beings have demonstrated how easily they can prosper on a wide range of foods. The right diet for you is an important and very personal choice, but no matter how carefully you choose, diet is only a small part of the total health equation.

In massage, diet and nutrition are considered separately. "You are what you eat." This mechanistic concept of nutrition might work if health were merely a question of consumption, but you can fill your stomach with the most nutritious food and do very little for your body.

The body receives no nutrition at all until food is digested and enters the bloodstream. At that point the nutritional requirements of the left foot depend on the quality of blood circulation to that foot and throughout its tissues. The most carefully planned diet will do almost nothing to develop important veins and arteries if it is not combined with vigorous exercise.

Unfortunately most exercise programs concentrate on a fraction of the body's 600 muscles. A tennis player will favor his racket arm. A runner may forget to develop his arms, and weight lifters often lack aerobic capacity. In every case when blood supply to the neglected area is reduced, *nutrition* is limited. Internal nutrition measures all the real benefits blood can bring to the body's tissues, including oxygen itself.

Massage can be used to boost internal nutrition rates that diet and exercise cannot affect. Masseurs can bring oxygen to overexercised muscles which are about to cramp or triple the blood supply to muscles that haven't been exercised at all. (See "Exercise and Massage," page 153.) Throughout the book you will find movements which are specifically designed to increase nutrition to parts of the body that most exercise programs ignore.

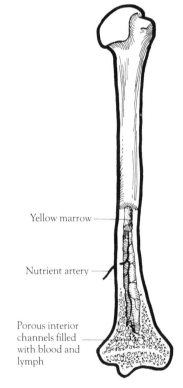

Yellow marrow

Nutrient artery

Porous interior channels filled with blood and lymph

Blood-soluble nutrients penetrate to all parts of a bone

The
Torso

The
Torso

The torso contains all of the body's vital organs except the brain. Since so many of the internal muscles around the organs are involuntary, your partner may not feel the immediate effects of massage. Nevertheless, the liver, lungs, and stomach all will benefit from movements in this chapter. The heart alone can be reached more effectively via certain nerves on the back. (see "Heart Massage," page 151). Massaging abdominal muscles, which are often underexercised, will definitely aid the digestive process. The kings of the Sandwich Islands were aware of this beneficial effect. They had themselves massaged after *every meal* to aid digestion. Do write if you find a restaurant that offers this delightful service. In the meantime, gourmet readers are encouraged to try light abdominal massage no more than one hour after a meal. Be sure to elevate your partner's torso with large pillows because lying flat just after eating puts a strain on the heart.

Massaging the abdomen stimulates blood circulation along the entire network of gastrointestinal veins and plays an important role in dispersing all body wastes. These wastes range from imperfectly digested food and lactic acid to the extremely fine tissue debris that is found throughout the body. The wastes serve as irritants until they are fully metabolized. Intestinal wastes that collect in the appendix are sometimes never properly metabolized. Perhaps someday the frequency of appendicitis in people who have received regular massage will be studied. I've never heard of a single such case.

The Front of the Legs

The Front of the Legs

The body's largest joint is also the most unpredictable one. Instead of acting like a simple hinge in the middle of a limb, the knee is constantly tempted to slide sideways, tearing internal ligaments, cartilage, and tendons. Each one of these injuries is sufficient to immobilize almost anyone. Many dancers and skiers end their careers with sudden knee injuries. Runners find themselves hardly able to walk, and people who avoid serious exercise to protect their knees can injure themselves while lifting a shopping bag. Knee injuries always seem to strike without warning. The only thing certain about them are the huge medical bills which always follow.

Must modern life become an inexorable journey from infancy to arthritis filled with giant knee pads and monster bandages? Since this is not a desirable (or fashionable) approach, the best alternative is to find ways to stabilize the naked knee. Masseurs who wish to consider this problem will do most of their work on the front of the leg. The four muscles that extend the knee joint and make it possible for you to rise from a chair are on the front of the thigh. All these parts connect to the knee via a single tendon. The kneecap actually grows out of the center of that tendon and many delicate internal parts of the knee are directly linked to this large four-sectioned muscle (called the quadriceps). If any part of the muscle is under- or overexercised, the knee is likely to suffer. Frequent massage will leave the quadriceps flexible and relaxed, the best possible state for healthy knee operation.

The Back of the Legs

The Back of the Legs

The sciatic nerve, one of the body's most important referred pain indicators, can be massaged on the back of the thigh. Pain here almost always indicates some sort of problem in the lower back and will serve as an important guide for you to plan your approach to the back itself.

Like headaches, lower back pain motivates millions of people to reach automatically for aspirin and other mildly addictive nonprescription drugs that knock out the whole nervous system. Massage proposes another route. Whenever possible in referred pain situations, begin by relaxing nerves around the site of the pain, and work back slowly to the source of the problem. Of course, there's no way to reach the center of the diaphragm after massaging its referred pain center at the top of the chest. But on the back of the leg you have an excellent opportunity to reach the sciatic nerve, its tributaries up and down the leg, and finally the lower back itself. There are three simple ways to isolate and detect sciatic nerve problems, and two of them work from the *front* of the leg. Pulling the leg and flexing the foot (see page 108) will almost always indicate sensitivity in the sciatic nerve area. The gluteus muscles that run across the buttocks and down onto the back of the legs have their insertion point on the front of the leg (see diagram, page 35). If, when you press around this insertion point, your partner feels shooting pains down the leg to the foot, you can be sure the sciatic nerve is irritated. The third point to check is toward the center of the thigh on the back of the leg. Right there the sciatic trunk is very close to the surface. Moderate pressure will usually tell you whether the nerve is going to require extra attention during your massage work on the back of the leg.

Nerve Percussion

thigh work best here. Your hands break contact one at a time to return to your partner's hip and stroke down to the knee.

Percussion can have either a stimulating or a sedative effect on a nerve. Mild superficial percussion movements will excite and awaken the nerves. If your partner complains of feeling sluggish and has been depending on large amounts of caffeine to get through the day, this is the sort of percussion that's called for as part of a general massage. But if the problem is pain, soreness, or irritation, you may want to use more pressure to relax the body. There's a kind of generally nervous temperament that keeps the nerves in a state of constant irritation. We all recognize "the overwrought, highly strung, nervous type, which is so commonly seen in the cities of the United States. Here life not only demands the most in human efficiency, but constantly keeps the nervous tensions high, whether it be in professional, commercial or social life. Even in athletics this tension is marked." [*]

Those words, written by an English masseuse, just after World War I, seem appropriately modern. Since she wrote, frantic attempts to solve this problem have produced the tranquilizer, an ominous little pill that forces people to relax (for a while) by inducing chemical changes in the brain. How much easier and safer to sedate the nerves with percussion movements that will not leave your partner depressed and anxiety-ridden a few hours later.

Nerve percussion is really a variation of slapping. By bending the ends of the fingers (as shown), you can direct the force of this movement so that specific nerves can be reached. It's not necessary to dig in with your fingertips. Your contact point should be around the fleshy balls of your fingertips. Like the other percussion movements, nerve percussion will flow more smoothly if you relax your hands and let them bend at the wrists. Work up and down the center of the leg three times.

[*] *Practical Massage and Corrective Exercises*, Nissen, op. cit.

Top-of-the-Leg Friction

Working from the top of the leg where muscle groups overlap around to the side (as shown), you can stimulate ligaments and tendons around the massive ball joint at the hip. The joint itself is off the center line of the leg bones toward the center of your partner's body. Working with friction movements, you can feel a depression at the side of the hip. There's plenty of room here for you to press inward and bring friction right up to the tissues around the joint. On this side of the leg, friction movements to the hip joint should move in a slow arc from the top center of the leg to the depression on the side of the hip and back again.

The Hip Press—A Passive Exercise

You can use the entire leg as a lever to exercise your partner's hip joint passively. This will work quite well as long as you remember to hold your partner's leg *above* the knee when you lift by grasping the lower part of the thigh. Be sure that no part of your hand presses against the delicate joint at the knee. Use your other hand to press down firmly (as shown) over the small part of the back. This will prevent your partner from rolling when you lift the leg and will maximize the movement you're creating at the hip joint. This movement is really limited by the flexibility of muscles on the front of the thigh. Working just to the point of tension, you can use it to stretch these muscles while you exercise the ball joint at the hip.

Kneading the Sides of the Leg

The inside: Since you don't have to avoid the femoral artery here, kneading pressures can be much greater than on the front of the leg. Don't be afraid to dig in with the full surface of both hands. Work up and down the leg three times—more if reducing is part of your partner's massage program. The thick hamstring muscles, used in walking, running, and dancing, almost always need toning during weight loss. Press down into them with your fingertips as you knead and be sure to use your thumbs. Knead all the way from the top of the leg to the foot, working in slow rhythmic circles. Pay special attention to the well defined muscles on the back of the knee. Stop there occasionally as you move up and down the leg and knead them with your fingertips. Runners and dancers will thank you for the extra care.

The outside: It's most comfortable to knead the outside of the leg the same way you kneaded the sides of the torso, from the opposite side of your partner's body (as shown). This movement

and it's a good idea to increase your pressure when you knead them. Again, pay special attention to the back of the knee.

will also provide an excellent transition when you're ready to move from one leg to another. You can do this by kneading up and down the inside of one leg, across the buttocks, and down the outside of the other leg. Stay in contact with the outside of the opposite thigh as you step across your partner's body to begin work on the leg. Tissues on the outside of the thigh are relatively firm

Knuckle Kneading

If your partner is in good shape and has been exercising regularly, you may find that the muscles on the back of the thigh seem hard even when they are relaxed. This is not necessarily a sign of tension but rather an indication that the body is not storing a great deal of surplus fat. Muscles that feel tight *under* a layer of fat are usually a sign that your partner is tense. As you work with massage, the difference between tense muscles and toned muscles becomes more readily apparent. You will usually find toned muscles on a fat-free, well-exercised body. They may feel tight, but only by comparison to muscles which are positively flabby.

If you can't find flesh to pick up with your thumb when you're kneading with the whole hand, it's time to try knuckle kneading. This movement allows you to exert much more pressure on the deep tissues of your partner's leg than fingertip or full-hand kneading. Press down evenly with the flat part of your knuckles (as shown). Rotate the hands in alternating circles the same way you would in any other kneading movement. Because the pressures are deep, you may want to add a bit more oil during this move-

Kneading the Buttocks

ment, particularly if your partner has hairy legs. Circle over the whole top of the thigh and onto the knee. Your right hand will always be down when your left hand is up.

Because they offer such a fine opportunity for kneading, the buttocks are always a great favorite with masseurs. If you're using massage along with exercise to help your partner lose weight, it's important to remember that many exercise programs unwittingly exclude these large muscles. The muscles of the buttocks will contract only against strong resistance like climbing stairs. Running and walking on level ground will not effectively tone them. Overweight runners who stubbornly refuse to recognize this fact begin to assume alarming pearlike shapes after a few weeks of running.

Knead the buttocks the same way you kneaded the sides of the legs: in long vertical motions. Depending on your partner's size, these kneading strokes may also include parts of the upper leg and lower back. Move slowly all the way across your partner's body over the buttocks. Work in parallel lines up and down the body, but when you reach the bony center, be careful not to press down on the spine. Buttock kneading allows you to pick up more flesh than any other kneading movement. Your partner will feel the difference when you cross over the entire center of the body, kneading deeply.

The Back

The Back

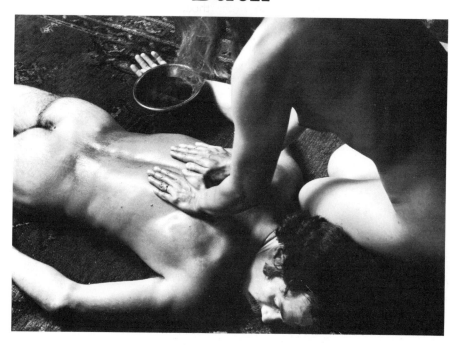

As a general (but by no means universal) rule, masseurs find that men and women experience tension in different parts of the body. Women are bothered by stiffness across the top of the back and at the base of the neck. Men complain of tension that develops into sharp pain around the lower back. People who suffer from aches and pains at either end of the back usually spend a lot of time worrying about it. Worrying tends to worsen the situation and create a vicious cycle since nervous anxiety may be causing the problem in the first place. This does not mean that the excruciating pain which strikes the lower back when something heavy is lifted improperly is imaginary. Rather, many sprains and muscle tears can be avoided if the back is massaged regularly. Internal tension, even in well-developed

muscles, reduces the range of response that is available to a relaxed muscle. By relaxing a muscle during massage, you restore its range of response and help protect your partner from similar accidents in the future.

Back problems, like circulatory diseases, are far more common now than they were 100 years ago. The sedentary middle-aged executive who suddenly breaks into a dead run while carrying three suitcases at the airport may also try lifting a refrigerator from a full standing position. People who live like this will soon find themselves far beyond the powers of any masseur. Almost any exercise program teaches one the limitations of the body. Intense back pain, particularly lower back pain, is definitely a signal that the body has been pushed beyond these limitations.

The Spine and the Nervous System

There are several signals which should be heeded before your partner actually tears the ligaments of the lower back or damages a disk. Some people complain of constant stiffness even after exercise. Others will take for granted persistent lower-back pain as a "normal" sign of aging. They may worry secretly about the pain while reminding themselves that back problems are unimportant. There is, however, no part of the body which is more crucial to an overall sense of well-being than the lower back. Since the spine itself is ultimately affected by muscle and nerve problems, it's always best to take lower-back complaints seriously. Deal with them promptly before they become nasty.

Almost nothing happens anywhere in the body without somehow involving the nervous system. Since the nervous system determines exactly how people will feel, relaxing it is the single most important concern in any full body massage. An hour of massage can have a spectacular effect on nervous people who have been dependent on the neighborhood drugstore for rest and relaxation. Dr. Douglas Graham, normally a conservative writer, described the effects of massage on his patient's nerves this way in his *Massage: Manual Treatment; Remedial Movements:*

Upon the nervous system, as a whole, massage most generally exerts a peculiarly delightful and at the same time profoundly sedative and tonic effect. While it is being done, and often for hours afterwards, the subjects are in a blissful state of repose; they feel as if they were enjoying a long rest . . . and quite frequently it makes optimists of them for the time being. An aptitude for rest or work usually follows, though generally those who submit to this treatment feel gloriously indifferent, and needless apprehensions are dispelled.

On the back, the body's main nerves are close to the surface and easily reached. By relaxing them, you can lower stress levels throughout the body and materially improve the health of every internal organ.

The nervous system is organized into a pattern that looks like an upside-down tree. Thirty-one pairs of spinal nerves branch out neatly across the back from the shoulders all the way down to the waist. These nerves supply all the internal organs and can be regarded as direct pathways to the interior of the body. At both ends of the back, other, longer branches spread out onto the limbs. Vertical nerves close to the spinal column control blood circulation, glands, and the crucial vasoconstriction response (see page 176). All these nerves form a massive communications network that connects directly to the 12 billion cells of the brain.

The spine is held erect and in place by two long groups of muscles that run parallel to it on both sides. If your partner is under a lot of pressure or just simply tense all the time, one of these muscle groups may become very tight. Not only is this tightness easily felt by a masseur,

How spinal nerves service the body

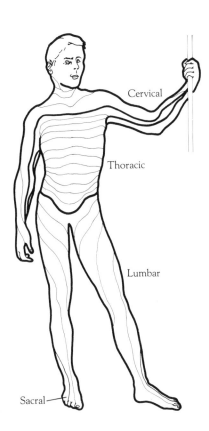

139

Two Super Relaxation Movements for the Back— Stroking Movements

but it is often actually visible. What you see are the muscles on one side of the spine pulling the spine and pinching nerves that supply the lower back and legs. The pain your partner feels may extend from the lower back right down the sciatic nerve onto one of the legs.

Although this sort of thing can be very painful, it's not necessarily that serious. If the doctor has decided that there's nothing wrong internally, you may find that back massage will bring your partner exactly the kind of immediate relief he craves.

If you want a simple way to introduce a friend to the joys of massage, try the following two movements twenty-five times each from both ends of the back. Between the two points you will reach every major muscle, nerve, and bone in the area. This 100-stroke sequence will leave your partner more relaxed than most two-week vacations.

The easiest, most balanced way of doing this stroke is by straddling your partner (as shown) and leaning forward with your whole body. Unless your partner is much smaller than you, it's OK to press down very hard as you move up the back. These are strong muscles; you won't overwhelm them. One thing you do want to avoid on the back, though, is direct pressure to the spine. With the exception of a few well-cushioned, very controlled movements, back massage works around the spine, not on it. Before you begin, make sure

you've oiled the whole back, including the shoulders and sides.

Press straight down on the base of your partner's back with the whole surface of both hands. You should just barely feel the edge of the spine between your fingers. Your hands follow the contour of your partner's body as it drops away from the spine. You will feel a smooth, even flesh contact from the base of your palms to the fingertips. The whole stroke moves up the back, maintaining this contact. Work all the way to the top of the back and out over the shoulders as you turn your hands. Pull down the sides of your partner's body, maintaining that full-hand contact. Pressures on the sides need not be as great as the ones you used going up the back. Pull all the way to the waist, and turn your hands so

Two Super Contact Movements That Use the Whole Forearm—Stroking Movements

These massive forearm movements are perfectly suited for the broad flat planes of the back. Depending on your partner's size, you can often cover the whole back from wrist to elbow without even moving your arm. Oiling both your forearms up to the elbow is lush and extravagant, but merely a suggestion of what your partner feels when you press both arms across the back. Keep your arms straight out and parallel until the very end of the arc is reached. You can usually press down quite hard while you move up and down the back.

Forearm compression will allow you to direct your pressures much more precisely. On the back, this movement works exactly the same way it did on the torso. Concentrate, once again, on the long muscles that parallel the spine. Remember to lower the flat part of your knuckles occasionally to maximize contact.

Flexing the Lower Back—A Passive Exercise

Here, again, is one of those rare massage movements in which physical strength is a factor. Unlike back cracking (see page 160), this passive exercise *can* be duplicated by your partner alone. Still, if size and strength permit, this is a fantastic addition to any back massage. Dancers absolutely crave it.

Gently slide your hands under your partner's shoulders, and grasp (as shown). Raise your outside leg, and plant the foot firmly. Lift your partner slowly, and as the torso rises, rest your elbow on the outstretched leg. This way your leg can act as a natural tripod to support your partner's body. Hold for a silent count of twenty, and lower your partner slowly and evenly.

Two Movements That Contact the Spine

Pressure on the spine means direct stimulation of the central nervous system. There are two ways this stimulation can affect your partner: You can either excite the nerves with brisk movements or sedate them with slow rhythmic strokes. If your partner has been depressed, quick movements up and down the spine will promote a feeling of exhilaration and well-being. If, on the other hand, you're dealing with insomnia, spasticity, nervousness, or hypertension, slow rhythmic strokes will produce a feeling of drowsiness and relaxation.

The closed-finger movement allows you to press down directly on top of the spine while the flesh of your hand cushions the contact. Although the fingertips are at the forward edge of this movement, you should actually lead with the base of your palm.

That's where the pressure is concentrated. The fingertips simply go along for the ride. Press down on your contact hand by crossing it (as shown) with your free hand. Reverse this movement at the shoulders, and move back to the waist without breaking contact or rhythm.

The open-finger contact movement moves up and down the back the same way. The difference is in the way pressures are distributed at your hands. The contact hand will touch your partner's back only at the fingertips and the base of the palm. The center of the hand and fingers remains arched throughout the movement. Try to equalize your contact pressure between the heel of your hand and the two contact fingers. The spine will fit neatly between the two contact fingers as you press up and down the back.

Heart Massage

Nerves that supply the heart branch off the spine between the shoulder blades. This is the area on which to concentrate if you want to soothe the heart. Two or three minutes of vigorous massage will usually reduce the pulse rate by about 10 percent. Vigorous, of course, does not mean violent. Work between the shoulder blades right up to the spine with friction, kneading, and vibration movements. The spine itself can be massaged with a combination of the two previous movements. A light percussion movement, like the hacking stroke you used on the leg (page 111), will nicely complement the sequence. Use it on the thick muscles around the spine, but stay off the spine itself. These movements will soothe the cardiac nerves and the heart muscle itself.

Down Stroking the Back

Pull down the spine with a hand-over-hand pressing movement. At the base of the spine bring your hands together so they merge into a ten-finger mandala (page 190). Concentrate on breaking this contact very slowly: with first the heel of the hand, then the palm, then the fingers, and finally the middle finger of the top hand, which should rest right on the spine. Move your hands up to your partner's shoulders one final time without touching his body. The hands are held just an inch above the skin during this final pass.

Massaging the Back of the Arm

When you're working on your partner's back, there's a whole range of movements you can get into on the back of the arms. The arms can be rotated (as shown), kneaded, and stroked from one end to another. You can certainly knead parts of the arm that were difficult, if not almost impossible, to reach from the other side of the body. Friction movements, particularly around the elbow, are very effective from this side of the body. You can, if you like, work out a whole sequence for the back of the arms. Be sure to duplicate all your movements on both arms and to give support, whenever you move an arm, above and below the elbow.

Completing a Massage

Use the full surface of your fingers to brush your partner's body from head to toes. At the toes final contact between ten fingertips and ten toes should be broken very slowly. Your partner will float up from that final moment as though his feet and body had actually left the ground. Mind and body merge at the end of a massage, and many people prefer not to be disturbed for some time. Withdraw from the massage area quietly. Be silent. Let the feeling go on.

152

Exercise and Massage

Exercise and Massage

People who exercise are usually very practical-minded and insist on knowing exactly what is going on inside the body. On one level they regard exercise as basic preventive medicine and constantly seek ways to make the machinery of the body work more efficiently. To this end, the overall effects of many health aids are sometimes very difficult to gauge. Diet changes, for example, can take months to register physically. The internal effects during and after massage, however, are immediate and apparent and have been measured.

A ten-minute abdominal massage will decrease, by as much as one hour, the decomposition time of food in the stomach. The assimilation rate of nutritious elements in the intestines rises significantly. This is particularly important to people who are fastidious about diet and want to get the greatest possible benefit from food. The whole digestive process is massively stimulated, and constipation can usually be dealt with quickly. Production of gastric juice, saliva, and urine is increased. Nitrogen, inorganic phosphorus, and sodium chloride levels in the urine are substantially higher. Many of these benefits have been observed one full week after a single, thorough body massage.

The Skin

Massage removes dead brittle skin from the surface and allows the living tissue beneath to breathe more easily. Tough, inflexible skin will become softer and far more supple after regular massage. Facial wrinkles, often merely the result of nervous tension, begin to disappear even if the face itself is not massaged. The effects of regular back massage, for example, will be apparent on the face. This is simply a result of the renewed vitality and overall health that massage can bring. Scalp massage stimulates the sebaceous secretion. Here again, the results are often actually visible. Afterward the hair looks glossy and moisturized.

Circulation and the Blood

Blood and lymph pass three times more rapidly through a part of the body being massaged than when it is not. While this happens, the pulse rate drops and the heart slows. Movements specifically intended to aid circulation momentarily empty the surface veins. Deep kneading strokes have a similar effect because the valves of the venous system will allow blood flow only toward the heart. Although these movements will speed local blood flow, their overall effect is to lower the blood pressure while they relax the heart and tone the vascular system. Massage cannot manufacture blood cells, but it can put into circulation those that are dormant in the body. Massage can be used to direct red and white blood corpuscles to specific parts of the body. Massive increases in the white blood cell count have been recorded after just five minutes of each of the following common movements: circulation, 85 percent; vibration and friction, 60 percent; percussion, 45 percent; and kneading, 30 percent. Enhanced blood supply will also act as a natural analgesic—that is, it will decrease pain. After massage the oxygen content of the tissues is up 10 to 15 percent, allowing for more efficient combustion of stored energy.

---

* Douglas Graham, M.D., *Massage: Manual Treatment; Remedial Movements*, J.B. Lippincott Company: Philadelphia, 1913, p. 83.

† Hermann Bucholz, *Therapeutic Exercise and Massage*, Lea & Febiger: Philadelphia and New York, 1920, p. 122.

The Muscles

Although the extraordinary Fluid Release effect was documented at the turn of the century, it has been ignored by antitactile societies for the past seven decades. Nevertheless, if you're interested in health, pay close attention to these astonishing ergographic tests which were designed to measure the work capacity of muscles before and after massage:

. . . *after severe exercise a rest of fifteen minutes brought about no essential recovery, whilst after massage for the same period the exercise was more than doubled. One person experimented upon lifted a weight of one kilo (2.2 pounds) eight hundred and forty times, at intervals of one second, by extreme flexion of the elbow-joint, from a table upon which the forearm rested horizontally, and after this he could do no more. When the arm had been massaged for five minutes, he lifted the weight more than eleven hundred times in the same manner as before without fatigue.* *

Professor Maggiora, of the University of Turin, has shown the restorative effects of massage upon his own muscles when weakened by physical or mental labor, by electricity, by hunger, loss of sleep, and slight fever. For this purpose the fatigue curves of the right and left middle fingers in maximum voluntary flexion were taken every two seconds with a weight of 3 kilograms. The average results showed that the muscles concerned in this movement could do about twice as much work after a few minutes of massage as they could without. †

The art of sensual
MASSAGE

Gordon Inkeles and Murray Todris

Touch and massage are an expression of sensuality. No special knack is needed. No great knowledge of anatomy or strange techniques. With only a warm, quiet place and a bottle of scented oil you can spread pleasure inch by inch, soothe away care, and imbue tranquility.

Sensitivity of touch can lend warmth to a new relationship or bring fresh life to a flagging one. It can bring intimacy to sex and sensuality to love.

The Art of Sensual Massage is written with a pleasant blend of friendliness and humour and warmth. Like massage it is something to enjoy at leisure, a book to browse through. It includes over 200 photographs and hints on oils and scents and erotic massage.

'Beautifully produced: a book to give, especially if you'd like its techniques used on you.'
Cosmopolitan

'Attractive as well as instructive . . . tells you what to massage, when and where. Much recommended.'
Forum

'If you want to encourage the man in your life to be more sensual, romantic and inventive . . . put *The Art of Sensual Massage* in his stocking.'
Miss London